Home Remedies

For Headaches

And Insomnia

Home Remedies
For Headaches
And Insomnia

By Monica Sidoine,
S.N.H.S. Dip. Herbalism

DISCLAIMER

This book is to serve as an informational guide for use in the home. The remedies and procedures contained in this book are meant to supplement and are not intended to be a substitute for professional medical care. Please seek a qualified medical practitioner for all ailments. The author nor distributors takes no responsibility for customers choosing to treat themselves. Your use of this information is at your own risk.

Copyright © 2016
By
Monica Sidoine

ISBN - 13: 978-1533580108
ISBN - 10: 1533580103

Proof Read by Jasmine Ned Anunda

Printed By Create Space Publishing
United States of America

ACKNOWLEDGMENTS

I would like to thank all those who have contributed in one way or another to the completion of HOME REMEDIES FOR HEADACHES AND INSOMNIA.

I thank God for giving me the vision, wisdom and good health to write this book. For all he has done and will continue to do in my life.

For the many prayer warriors who interceded on behalf of this project and also their moral support.

I thank my daughter Jasmine Ned Anunda for proof reading.

Thank you all.

Monica Sidoine.

PREFACE

The procedures in this Book was designed to be as simple as possible so that anyone will be able to follow them. Most of the items used are local things which you would either have at home, in your kitchen garden or can be easily purchased from the local market or health store for a very low cost.

TABLE OF CONTENTS

Acknowledgements 5

Preface...7

Headaches 10

Cluster Headaches 15

Congestive Headaches 17

Migraine 18

Tension Headaches 22

Insomnia 24

Hydrotherapy Treatments 30

HEADACHES

A headache is a pain in the head lasting for some time, caused by changes in pressure in the blood vessels leading to and from the brain.

Some common causes are:-

Stress, tension, colds, fevers, eye ache, allergies, menstruation, and constipation.

There can be many causes of a headache such as:-

Physiological changes in the head, constriction of blood vessels, abnormal neuron activity, genetic causes, excessive smoking, excessive drinking of alcohol, lack of water in the body, oversleeping, lack of sleep, overuse of pain killers, eye strain, neck strain, sinus, migraine, long time exposure to sun, tiredness, hunger, skipped meals, poor body posture, changes in season, lack of a nutritious diet, certain fragrances or smell, certain hair accessories like tight-fitting hair bands, hats, etc., hormonal changes and having ice-creams.

Some of the symptoms are:-

Dull ache affecting entire head, pain during sleep which lasts for at least 90 minutes, throbbing sensation, sensitivity to sound and light, vomiting or nausea, redness of eye, loss of appetite, nasal congestion, fever and dizziness, unclear vision and fatigue; constant pain in forehead, cheekbones and bridge of the nose.

NATURAL REMEDIES

- Boil 1oz of red clover in 1 liter of water for 30 minutes.
  Drink one cup when the headache comes on.

- Boil 1oz of ginger in 1 liter of water for 20 minutes.
  Drink 1 cup twice daily.

- Steep 1oz each of crushed rosemary leaves and crushed sage
  leaves in 1 liter of boiling water.
  Drink 1 cup three times daily.

- Steep 1oz of feverfew in 1 liter of boiling water for 30
  minutes.
  Drink 1 cup twice a day.

- Steep 1oz of basil leaves in 1 liter of boiling water for 30
  minutes.
  Drink 1 cup twice a day.

- Steep 1oz of sage leaves in 1 liter of boiling water for 30
  minutes.
  Drink 1 cup three times daily.

- Steep 10 neem leaves in 4 cups of boiling water for 30
  minutes.
  Drink one cup three times daily.

- Mix 2 tablespoons each of ginger juice and lemon juice.
  Take it once daily.

- Add 1 tablespoon of sugar to a glass of watermelon juice. Drink it daily.

- Chew 1 or 2 pieces of crystallized ginger candy.

- Eat two neem leaves daily.

- Eat two basil leaves daily.

- Use spinach leaves as part of your salad.

- Eat some raw pumpkin seeds.

- Eat raw cabbage and several stalks of raw celery.

- Use cayenne powder in your cooking.

- Sprinkle a pinch of salt on an apple.
  Eat it every day on an empty stomach.

- Blend the juice of one lemon or orange with 2 tablespoons of sesame seeds.

- Mix 3 drops of peppermint essential oil in 1 tablespoon of almond or coconut oil.
  Massage your forehead, temples and the back of the jaws with it.

- Mix 3 drops of rosemary oil in 1 tablespoon of almond or coconut oil.
  Massage your forehead and temples with it.

- Put a few drops of lavender essential oil on the forehead.

- Bring the thumb and index finger close together. Press and massage the fleshy area between them at the highest spot of the muscle. Do it for 2 minutes and then repeat on the other hand.

Note: Do not press this acupressure point during pregnancy.

- Crush some fresh peppermint or coriander leaves and put it on your forehead.

- Mix some cinnamon with water to make a paste.
  Apply it all over the forehead.

- Make a paste of 1 teaspoon of ginger powder and 2 tablespoons of water.
  Apply it all over the forehead for a few minutes.

- Get a full body massage.

- Exercise daily for at least 30 minutes.

- Do some deep breathing exercises.

- Have at least 8 hours of sleep nightly.

- Relax for 10 minutes in a dark room with your eyes closed.

- Moisten 2 peppermint or chamomile tea bags.
  Place 1 over each eyelid for at least 10 minutes.

- Place a washcloth dipped in ice-cold water over the head for 5 minutes.
  Repeat it several times.

- Boil 1oz of ginger in 1 liter of water.
  Use it as a steam inhalation.
  See the Hydrotherapy Section.

- Add a few drops of peppermint or lavender essential oil to the water for a steam inhalation.
  See the Hydrotherapy Section

- Hot foot bath.
  See the Hydrotherapy Section.

- Take a hot water shower or bath.

Health Tips

- Reduce the stress in your life.

- Simplify your life.

- Practice aerobic activities, like swimming, biking, and walking.

- Avoid smoking.

- Avoid intake of nitrites and nitrates.

- Eat the right food.

- Stay calm and positive.

- Avoid dairy products, chocolates and pickles.

- Get plenty of sleep.

- Avoid strain on eyes.

- Avoid alcohol consumption, red wine and caffeine.

- Stay hydrated.

- Avoid artificial sweeteners.

CLUSTER HEADACHES

A severe recurring headache associated with the release of histamine in the blood stream and marked by sudden sharp pain behind one eye or nostril. The pain lasts for one to two hours on average and may recur several times in a day.

Causes and symptoms are:-

Biochemical, hormonal, and vascular changes induce cluster headaches, but why these changes occur remains unclear.

Episodic cluster headaches seem to be linked to changes in day length, possibly signaling a connection to the so-called biological clock.

Alcohol, tobacco, histamine, or stress can trigger cluster headaches. Decreased blood oxygen levels (hypoxemia) can also act as a trigger, particularly during the night when an individual is sleeping. Interestingly, the triggers do not cause cluster headaches during remission periods.

The primary cluster headache symptom is excruciating one-sided head pain centered behind an eye or near the temple. This pain may radiate outward from the initial focus and encompass the mouth and teeth. For this reason, some cluster headache sufferers may mistakenly attribute their pain to a dental problem.

Secondary symptoms, occurring on the same side as the pain, include eye tearing, nasal congestion followed by a runny nose, pupil contraction, and facial drooping or flushing.

NATURAL REMEDIES

- Put 1 heaping teaspoonful of cayenne pepper in 2oz of rubbing alcohol. Shake vigorously 3 times a day for 3 days. Let it settle and use the liquid from the top. Put 2 drops into an ounce of normal saline (make it by putting a level teaspoon of salt into a pint of water), and shake well.

VERY CAREFULLY put several drops of this mixture into the nostril that is involved, holding the head back. If you have a nasal sprayer, one spray is sufficient.
Do this 6 times a day for 6 days.
If the headaches are still on do it 3 times a day until they are gone. If the solution is too hot to tolerate, dilute it in half with the normal saline and try again. If headaches continue, repeat the course as needed.

N.B. It will burn but wears off within a few minutes.

Health Tips

- Avoid anything which will trigger the headache.

- Take heed to medical treatment.

- Avoid dust, smoke, perfume.

- Try to control any stress which maybe in your life currently.

CONGESTIVE HEADACHES

Headaches which occur when the sinuses become infected, inflamed or obstructed. If there is a cold, sinus problems, allergies and nasal congestion.

NATURAL REMEDIES

- Steep 1oz of sage in 1 liter of boiling water for 30 minutes. Drink 1 cup twice a day.

- Steep 1oz of peppermint in 1 liter of boiling water for 30 minutes.
  Drink 1 cup twice daily.

- Boil 1oz of cinnamon in 1 liter of boiling water for 15 minutes.
  Drink 1 cup twice daily.

- Make a paste with crushed cinnamon bark and a little water added to it.
  Apply it to the forehead.

- Place a washcloth soaked with sage tea over the painful part of the head.

- Steep 1oz of chamomile, rosemary or parsley in 1 liter of boiling water for 30 minutes.
  Use it as an eye compress.
  See the Hydrotherapy Section.

MIGRAINE

Migraine is a recurrent throbbing, very painful headache, often affecting one side of the head and sometimes accompanied by vomiting, or by distinct warning signs including visual disturbances.

It starts with a mild to moderate pain and then turn severe.

Some causes are food allergies, stress, tension, not enough exercise, menstruation, toothache and low blood sugar.

NATURAL REMEDIES

- Steep 1oz of feverfew in 1 liter of boiling water for 30 minutes.
  Drink 1 cup twice a day.

- Steep 1oz of peppermint in 1 liter of boiling water for 30 minutes.
  Drink 1 cup four times daily.

- Steep 1oz of basil leaves or oregano in 1 liter of boiling water for 30 minutes.
  Drink 1 cup four times daily.

- Steep 1oz of rosemary in 1 liter of boiling water for 30 minutes.
  Drink ½ cup three times daily.

- Steep 1oz of lemon grass in 1 liter of boiling water for 30 minutes.
  Drink 1 cup four times daily.

- Steep 1oz of chamomile in 1 liter of boiling water for 30 minutes.
  Drink 1 cup four times daily.

- Steep 6 orange leaves or 9 lemon leaves in 1 liter of boiling water for 30 minutes.
  Drink 4 cups daily.

- Take two teaspoons of honey before each meal.

- Have some sesame seeds along with your meal.

- Eat lots of raw onions and garlic.

- At the start of a migraine, put 5 - 10 drops of cayenne extract in the nostril on the side of the headache. Hold it in the nostril.
  The headache is usually gone in about 10 minutes. If the headache has been on for a while put it in both sides of the nostril.

  Cayenne Extract: Put ¼ teaspoon of cayenne pepper in one cup of pure grain alcohol. Let it set for two days and strain or pour off the top portion.

- Bend the head forward, pour 1 quart of ice water on the scalp at the nape of the neck for 1 minute. Let it flow under the hair to the forehead to drip. Pour 1 quart of ice water over the feet for 1 minute. Dry both the scalp and feet and rest.

- Take a hot foot bath with a cold compress or ice pack over the painful area.
  See the Hydrotherapy Section.

- Put both feet in very hot water for 2 minutes only.
  Dry the feet quickly and rest.

N.B. Do not do this treatment for diabetics.

- Garlic foot bath.
  Do it for ½ an hour daily.
  See the Hydrotherapy Section.

N.B. Do not do this treatment for diabetics.

- Apply a cold compress to the head with small chips of ice in the cold towel or an ice pack to the forehead.

- Place a washcloth dipped in ice-cold water over the head for 5 minutes.
  Repeat it several times.

- Apply an ice pack to the back of your neck.

- Wet a sock in one area with vinegar. Put the vinegar part over the painful area and pin it around the head.

- A Steam Inhalation for 10 minutes 3 times daily until better.
  Add 1 drop of basil oil or 2 drops of lavender essential oil in the water.
  See the Hydrotherapy Section.

- Boil equal parts of honey and vinegar.
  Use it as a Steam Inhalation.
  See the Hydrotherapy Section.

- Put 3 drops of lavender essential oil on a tissue and inhale it.

- Mix 1 part of rosemary oil in 10 parts of coconut oil.
  Rub it on the temples and the forehead.

- Mix 3 drops of lavender essential oil in 1 tablespoon of coconut or almond oil.
  Massage the forehead with it.

- Mix 1 tablespoon of garlic oil in one pint of rubbing alcohol. Rub it across the forehead.

Garlic Oil: Heat 1oz olive oil and 3 cloves of crushed garlic for about 3 minutes, strain and bottled for when ready to use. 3 drops of eucalyptus oil or glycerin can be added to help preserve it. Store in the refrigerator for when ready to use.

- Rub the neck and shoulders with vinegar.

Health Tips

- Avoid using dairy products.

- Avoid using chocolate.

- Avoid using white sugar.

- Avoid using fried foods.

- Avoid using alcoholic drinks.

- Avoid using shellfish.

TENSION HEADACHES

Can cause pain in the head, neck and behind the eyes, usually associated with muscle tightness.

NATURAL REMEDIES

- Simmer 4 fresh basil leaves in 2 cups of boiling water for a few minutes.
  Sip it slowly.

- Chew some fresh basil leaves.

- Put a few ice cubes in a plastic bag with a little water. Apply it to the neck and upper back for 10 minutes. Then apply warm towels or heating pads for 60 minutes.

- Apply hot avocado leaves to the forehead.

- Crush some cloves and add a little water to make a paste. Apply it on the forehead.

- Mix 2 drops of clove oil in a tablespoon of coconut or almond oil.
  Massage your forehead and temples with it.

- Mix 2 drops of basil oil with 2 drops of coconut oil. Massage your forehead with it.

- Mix together 2 teaspoons of coconut oil, 1 teaspoon of sea salt and 2 drops of clove oil.
  Massage it on your forehead.

- Mix 2 drops of coconut oil with 2 drops of lavender or rosemary essential oil.
  Apply it to the back of the neck and the forehead.

- Garlic foot bath.
  Use it as a Cold Footbath for 3 minutes daily.
  See the Hydrotherapy Section.

- Do a Steam Inhalation and add 2 drops of eucalyptus or lavender essential oil.
  See the Hydrotherapy Section.

- Boil 1 tablespoon of basil leaves in 1 liter of water or a few drops of basil oil added to it.
  Use it for a Steam Inhalation.
  See the Hydrotherapy Section.

- Crush a few cloves gently and put them in a cotton cloth and inhale it.

- Put 3 drops of eucalyptus oil on a washcloth and inhale.

- Put 3 drops of lavender essential oil on a tissue and inhale it.

- Coconut Oil Pack.
  See the Hydrotherapy Section.

- Exercise for at least 30 minutes daily.

- Avoid sugar and caffeine.

INSOMNIA

Insomnia is the inability to fall asleep or to remain asleep long enough to feel rested, especially when this is a problem that continues overtime.

Insomnia is generally of two types: - Acute and Chronic.

Acute insomnia is usually more common and lasts for days or weeks.

Chronic insomnia, on the other hand, lasts for months or even longer.

This leads to daytime fatigue, poor performance, tension headaches, irritability, depression, and various other problems.

Some causes are:-

Having a heavy meal just before bedtime and overeating, going to bed hungry. Also disorders in the brain, digestive system, lungs, endocrines, liver and heart. Stress, anxiety, depression, psychotic disorders, poor sleep habits, disruptions in sleeping environment, frequent naps during day, disturbing sleep events like nightmares, sleep walking, restless leg syndrome, life changes, changes in work shift, caffeine or other stimulants, smoking, aging, chronic pain, breathing difficulties, and certain medical conditions such as arthritis, heart failure, acid reflux, impact of medications, traumatic injury, fear or phobia, and frequent urination due to diabetes are some of the common causes that contribute to insomnia.

It can also be a side effect of certain medications such as corticosteroids, alpha-blockers, beta-blockers, ACE inhibitors, and more.

NATURAL REMEDIES

- Steep ½oz of chamomile in 2 cups of boiling water for 30 minutes.
  Drink 1 cup twice a day.

- Steep 1oz of peppermint in 1 liter of boiling water for 30 minutes.
  Drink 1 cup 3 times daily.

- Steep 1oz of red rose petals in 1 Liter of boiling water for 15 minutes. It can be sweetened with honey.
  Drink 4-6 cups daily.

- Steep 2oz of lettuce in 2 pints of boiling water for 10 minutes.
  Drink 2 large cups sweetened with a teaspoon of honey 1 hour before bedtime.

- Steep 6 orange leaves to 1 liter of boiling water for 30 minutes.
  Drink 4 cups daily, the last one just before bedtime.

- Steep 1oz of lemon leaves in 1 liter of boiling water for 30 minutes.
  Drink 4 cups daily.

- Steep 1oz of passion fruit leaves and flowers in 1 liter of boiling water for 3 minutes.
  Drink 4 cups daily. The last one just before bedtime.

- Steep 1oz of sage in 1 liter of boiling water for 30 minutes. Drink 1 cup three times daily.

- Boil 1 teaspoon of cumin seeds in 2 cups of water for 4 minutes.
  Drink it at bedtime.

- Simmer 1 teaspoon of aniseeds in 2 cups of water for 10 minutes. Strain it. Add ½ tablespoon of honey and ¼ cup of milk.
  Sip it daily just before bedtime.

- Steep 9 soursop leaves in 1 liter of boiling water for 30 minutes.
  Drink 4 cups daily, the last one at bedtime.

- Stir 1 tablespoon of honey and ¼ teaspoon of nutmeg in 8oz of hot milk. Allow it to cool a little.
  Drink it half an hour before bedtime.

- Stir 1 tablespoon of honey and ¼ teaspoon of cinnamon powder in 8oz of hot milk. Allow it to cool a little.
  Drink it half an hour before bedtime.

- Steep ½ teaspoon of saffron in a cup of warm milk.
  Drink it before bedtime.

- Stir ¼ teaspoon of cinnamon powder in a cup of warm milk.
  Drink it one hour before bedtime.

- Stir ¼ teaspoon of nutmeg in 1 cup of warm water or any fruit juice.
  Drink it before bedtime.

- Drink a hot fresh lemon drink first thing in the morning and last thing at night.

- Drink a banana smoothie at least 1 hour before bedtime.

- Stir 2 teaspoons of honey in 1 cup of water.
  Take it daily.

- Take a spoonful of honey just before bedtime.

- Extract 2 teaspoons of juice from fenugreek leaves and add 1 teaspoon of honey to it.
  Take it daily.

- Extract the juice from crushed celery leaves and the stalk.
  Mix 1 tablespoon of the juice with 1 tablespoon of honey.
  Take it at night.

- Mash 1 ripe banana and combine it with 1 teaspoon of cumin powder.
  Eat it before going to bed.

- Eat a few mandarins after dinner in the evening.
  It has bromine which is sedative to the nervous system.

- Steep sesame seeds for 20 minutes. Strain and toast lightly.
  Take two teaspoons after breakfast and lunch.

- Have oatmeal with 2 tablespoons of flaxseed added to it.

- Eat toast, banana and peanut butter.

- Eat 4oz of almonds daily.

- Consume raw onion salad.

- Eat lots of oats, lettuce, tomato, potato, pepper and eggplant.

- Sprinkle a few drops of lavender oil on the pillow just before going to sleep.

- Spread some basil leaves around the corners of the bed and under the pillow to inhale the smell.

- Apply a few drops of jasmine oil to the wrist just before bedtime.

- Apply a few drops of lavender oil to the forehead and temples just before bedtime.

- Massage your toes with milk just before bedtime.

- Massage your feet with sesame oil just before bedtime.

- Get a full body massage at least twice weekly.

- Have a warm bath just before bedtime with a few drops of either chamomile, rosemary or lavender essential oil added to it. Relax for 10 minutes in it.

- Garlic foot bath.
  Use it for half an hour daily.
  Put in the hot bath for 3 minutes and then in the cold bath for 1 minute ending with the cold bath.
  See the Hydrotherapy Section.

- Have a 1 hour brisk walk during the day and a walk or gentle stretching exercises after the evening meal.

- Try to get at least 20 minutes of sunlight daily.

- **For infants:** Soak in a hot water bath for three minutes.

Health Tips

- Perform deep breathing exercises and meditation.

- Sleep in a peaceful, dark and comfortable room.

- Try to have your last meal at least 4-5 hours before bedtime.

- Listen to soft music around 45 minutes before going to bed.

- Avoid watching TV before bedtime.

- Avoid the consumption of alcohol and caffeine.

- Avoid naps during the day time.

- Do not take any tea, cola drinks, alcohol, coffee or cigarettes after 5 p.m. Take herbal teas instead.

- Do not eat any meat.

- Do not eat any chocolate.

- Do not eat any cheese.

- Do not eat any ham.

- Stay away from laptop, iPod, and smart phones at night, they reduce the secretion of melatonin.

HYDROTHERAPY TREATMENTS

COCONUT OIL PACKS

An oil soaked cloth usually hot and placed over the abdomen.

Will assist in elimination, good for headaches and constipation.

Items needed:

Coconut oil
Cotton flannel cloth
Plastic sheet
Bath towel
Two safety pins
Hot water bottle

Method:

Fold the flannel in two layers wide and long enough to cover and wrap around the area if need to. Soak the flannel with warm coconut oil but not dripping. Put it on the abdomen, cover with the plastic. Wrap a towel around the area and fasten it with safety pins. A hot water bottle can be placed on it. Leave it on for at least 8 hours. Wash off with 2 teaspoons of baking soda to 1 quart of water. Use it every day with one day off each week and week 4 off, it can be repeated until improvement.

GARLIC FOOT BATH

Procedure:

Crush 5 garlic cloves and pour ¾ gallons of boiling water over it. Cover and steep for half day. Heat it and then strain. Use it as a footbath for 30 minutes daily. Put the feet in the hot bath for 3 minutes and then in the cold bath for 1 minute ending with the cold bath. Repeat 7 times.

COLD COMPRESS

Dip a washcloth in a basin with ice and cold water. Squeeze out the excess water. Fold and lay it on the area to be treated. Pieces of ice can be put in the fold. Change the washcloth every 3 minutes wiping the area often with a cold cloth until relief is obtained. Dry thoroughly at the end of the treatment. It can be applied to any part of the body especially the face, forehead and neck.

Contraindications:

Do not use if the person have sinus or pleurisy.
Do not use it on a chilled person.

EYE COMPRESS

This treatment helps acute glaucoma, acute iridocyclitis, sties, eye irritation and burning.

N.B. This treatment is to be used as first aid. Please see an eye specialist.

Method:

1. Put some cotton in the scoop section of a long wooden spoon, wrap it with cotton cloth and tie it.
2. Dip it in hot water and squeeze the excess water.
3. Apply it to the eye for 20 minutes every three hours.

HOT FOOT BATH

It is very good for headaches, colds, flu, coughs, congestion, nosebleed, earache, sinusitis, menstrual pains, fatigue, fever, pelvic cramps and congestion, prostate disorders, nervous tension, toothaches, backaches, infections, relaxation, stimulates circulation and warms the body.

Items needed:

1 bucket about quarter filled with hot water.
Small basin of ice water.
Large pan of very hot water.
2 washcloths for the head compress.
1 sheet and a blanket or 2 sheets.
1 hand towel for the neck.
1 bath towel.
1 bath mat.

Procedure:

1. Drape a blanket to completely cover a chair, then cover the blanket with a sheet.
2. Place a bucket ¼ filled with hot water on a bath mat in front of the chair.
3. Remove clothing, sit and wrap with the sheet, then the blanket.
4. Close all doors and windows.
5. Place the feet into the bucket and wrap the sheet and blanket around the bucket to avoid the circulation of air.
6. Wrap a hand towel around the neck to hold the sheet and blanket in place.
7. Apply a cold compress to the forehead, changing it every 3 minutes.
8. Maintain the water temperature in the bucket by adding more hot water continuously by pushing the persons feet to one side and placing your hands as a shield between the feet and the flow of hot water.
9. Continue adding the hot water for 20-30 minutes or an hour if needed. When sweating begins give the person water to drink at intervals throughout the treatment.

10. At the end of the treatment lift the feet up and pour cold water over them very quickly, dry and put on warm socks. Unwrap and dry the body. Dress, cover warmly and rest for 30-60 minutes. Take a cool shower.

A heating pad placed on the lower abdomen and upper thighs or a heating compress on the feet repeated every 4 hours can be used to replace the hot foot bath.

N.B. Do not use this treatment for persons with diabetes, loss of feelings, unconscious, arteriosclerosis, elevated pulse.

STEAM INHALATION

Effects:

1. Relieves nasal and lung congestions.
2. Relieves coughs.
3. Secretions are loosen and it is easier to expectorate.
4. Blood flow is increased to the throat and lungs.
5. Relieves sinus headaches.

Contraindications:

1. Persons suffering with congestive heart failure.
2. Persons suffering with asthma.

Items needed:

Basin with boiling water
Umbrella and sheet
Bedside stand and chair
A few drops of wintergreen or eucalyptus oil,
or 1 teaspoon Vicks VapoRub, or 2 tablespoons of herbs.

Procedure:

1. Fill a face basin with boiling water and add medication or herb if desired.
2. Put it on a table or bedside stand. Sit on a chair and open an umbrella over the head then cover with a sheet to form a tent over the head and basin. Instead of the umbrella and sheet, a large thick towel can be used to cover the head and basin.
3. Inhale the steam for 30 to 60 minutes 2 – 3 times daily.
4. Dry the face and any other moist areas of the body.
5. Rest for half an hour.

Other Book Titles by the Same Author

Can be viewed at this link:
http://www.amazon.com/author/monicasidoine

Home Remedies For Cancer

Home Remedies For Losing Weight

Home Remedies For Blood Pressure and Diabetes

Home Remedies For Stress, Depression and Anxiety

Home Remedies For Sinusitis and Tonsillitis

Home Remedies For Constipation and Diarrhea

Home Remedies For Asthma and Bronchitis

Home Remedies For Dehydration and Vomiting

Home Remedies For Pneumonia and Tuberculosis

NOTES

NOTES

NOTES

NOTES